Plant-Base Meals for Beginners

The Most Complete Collection of Super-Easy Recipes to Boost Your Diet and Save Time

||| | ||||||||||| |||| ||||| ||| |||| ||| |||
I0145883

Dave Ingram

Table of contents

Pea Salad

Preparation Time: 40 minutes

Cooking Time: 0 minute

Servings: 6

Ingredients:

1 cup chickpeas, rinsed and drained 1 ½ cups peas, divided

Salt to taste

3 tablespoons olive oil

½ cup buttermilk Pepper to taste

8 cups pea greens 3 carrots, shaved

1   cup snow peas, trimmed

Directions:

1.   Add the chickpeas and half of the peas to your food processor.

2.   Season with salt.

3.   Pulse until smooth. Set aside.

4.   In a bowl, toss the remaining peas in oil, milk, salt, and pepper.

5.   Transfer the mixture to your food processor.

6.   Process until pureed.

7.   Transfer this mixture to a bowl.

8.   Arrange the pea greens on a serving plate.

9.   Top with the shaved carrots and snow peas.

10.   Stir in the pea and milk dressing.

11.   Serve with the reserved chickpea hummus.

Nutrition:

Calories: 214 Fat: 8.6g Carbs: 27.3g Protein: 8g

Snap Pea Salad

Preparation Time: 1 hour

Cooking Time: 0 minute

Servings: 6

Ingredients:

2   tablespoons mayonnaise

¾ teaspoon celery seed

¼ cup cider vinegar

1 teaspoon yellow mustard 1 tablespoon sugar

Salt and pepper to taste

4 oz. radishes, sliced thinly

12 oz. sugar snap peas, sliced thinly

Directions:

1.   In a bowl, combine the mayonnaise, celery seeds, vinegar, mustard, sugar, salt, and pepper.

2.   Stir in the radishes and snap peas.

3.   Refrigerate for 30 minutes.

Nutrition:

Calories: 69 Fat: 3.7g Carbs: 7.1g Protein: 2g

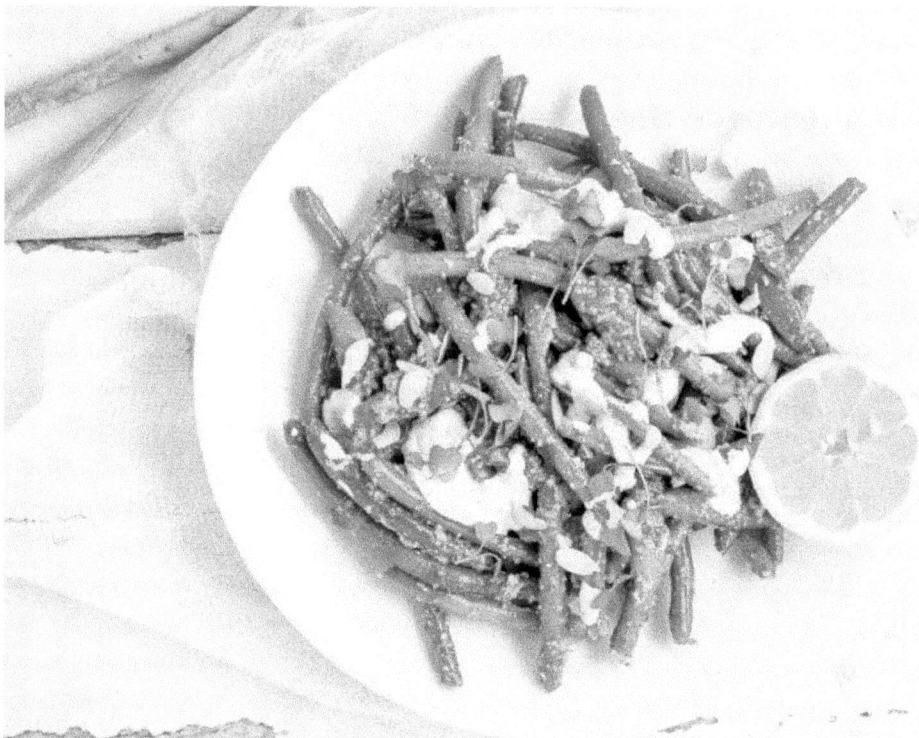

Cucumber Tomato Chopped Salad

Preparation Time: 15 minutes

Cooking Time: 0 minute

Servings: 6

Ingredients:

½ cup light mayonnaise 1 tablespoon lemon juice

1 tsp fresh dill

1 tbsp chives, chopped

½ cup feta cheese, crumbled Salt and pepper to taste

1 red onion, chopped 1 cucumber, diced

1 radish, diced

3 tomatoes, diced Chives, chopped

Directions:

1.   Combine the mayo, lemon juice, fresh dill, chives, feta cheese, salt, and pepper in a bowl. Mix well.

2.   Stir in the onion, cucumber, radish, and tomatoes. Coat evenly.

3.   Garnish with the chopped chives.

Nutrition:

Calories: 187 Fat: 16.7g Carbs: 6.7g Protein: 3.3g

Zucchini Pasta Salad

Preparation Time: 4 minutes

Cooking Time: 0 minute

Servings: 15

Ingredients:

5 tablespoons olive oil

2   teaspoons Dijon mustard

3   tbsp red-wine vinegar

1 garlic, grated

2 tablespoons fresh oregano, chopped

1 shallot, chopped

¼ teaspoon red pepper flakes 16 oz. zucchini noodles

¼ cup Kalamata olives pitted

3 cups cherry tomatoes, sliced in half

¾ cup Parmesan cheese shaved

Instructions:

1.   Mix the olive oil, Dijon mustard, red wine vinegar, garlic, oregano, shallot, and red pepper flakes in a bowl.

2.   Stir in the zucchini noodles.

3.   Sprinkle on top the olives, tomatoes, and Parmesan cheese.

Nutrition:

Calories: 299 Fat: 24.7g Carbs: 11.6g Protein: 7g

Egg Avocado Salad

Preparation Time: 10 minutes

Cooking Time: 0 minute

Servings: 4

Ingredients:

1 avocado

6 hard-boiled eggs, peeled and chopped 1 tablespoon mayonnaise

2 tablespoons freshly squeezed lemon juice

¼ cup celery, chopped

2 tablespoons chives, chopped Salt, and pepper to taste

Instructions:

1.   Add the avocado to a large bowl.

2.   Mash the avocado using a fork.

3.   Stir in the egg and mash the eggs.

4.   Add the mayo, lemon juice, celery, chives, salt, and pepper.

5.   Put in the fridge for 23 minutes before serving.

Nutrition:

Calories: 224 Fat: 18g Carbs: 6.1g Protein: 10.6g

Pepper Tomato Salad

Preparation Time: 1 hour and 25 minutes

Cooking Time: 0 minute

Servings: 8

Ingredients:

2 tablespoons balsamic vinegar 2 tablespoons olive oil

½ teaspoon Dijon mustard

2 teaspoons fresh basil leaves, chopped 1 tablespoon fresh chives, chopped

1   teaspoon sugar Pepper to taste

2   cups yellow bell peppers, sliced into rings 1 cups orange bell pepper, sliced into rings 4 tomatoes, sliced into rounds

¼ cup blue cheese, crumbled

Instructions:

1.　　Mix the vinegar, olive oil, mustard, basil, chives, sugar, and pepper in a bowl.

2.　　Arrange the tomatoes and pepper rings on a serving plate.

3.　　Sprinkle the crumbled blue cheese on top.

4.　　Drizzle with the dressing.

5.　　Chill in the refrigerator for 1 hour before serving.

Nutrition:

Calories: 116 Fat: 7g Carbs: 11g Protein: 3g

Potato Mash

Preparation Time: 10 minutes

Cooking Time: 9 minutes

Servings: 6

Ingredients:

1 and 1/2 pounds white potatoes, peeled, chopped 1 teaspoon salt

1/2 teaspoon hot paprika 1 teaspoon dill, dried

1 tablespoon coconut butter

1 teaspoon ground black pepper 1 cup vegetable broth

1 tablespoon fresh parsley, chopped

Directions:

1.   Put potatoes, salt, and vegetable broth in the instant pot.

2.   Close the lid and set manual mode. Cook on High for 9 minutes.

3.   Then make quick pressure release, strain the sweet potatoes and mash until smooth.

4.   Stir well and serve.

Nutrition: Calories: 123, Fat: 4.3, Fiber: 2.2, Carbs: 11.4, Protein: 4.3

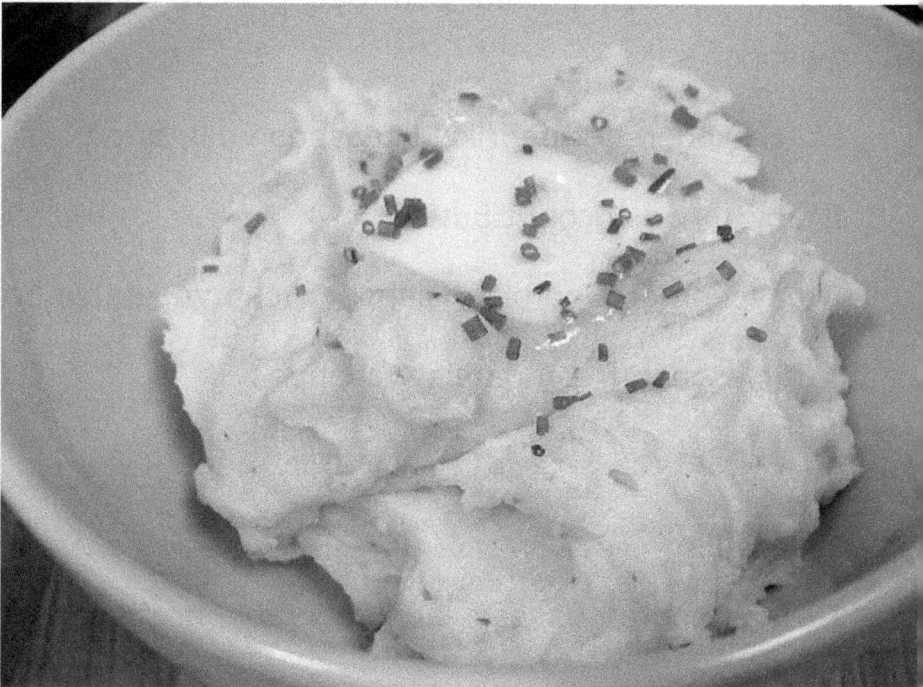

Red Cabbage and Carrots

Preparation Time: 10 minutes

Cooking Time: 7 minutes

Servings: 3

Ingredients:

1-pound red cabbage, shredded 2 carrots, peeled and grated

1 tsp powder

1 tsp coriander, ground 1 teaspoon black pepper

1   teaspoon salt

1/4 cup of coconut milk 3/4 cup almond milk

1/2 tablespoon chives, chopped

Directions:

1.   In the instant pot, mix the cabbage with the carrots and the other ingredients, toss and set manual mode (High pressure).

2.   Cook the cabbage for 7 minutes. Then allow natural pressure release.

3.   Transfer the meal into the serving bowls and cool down before serving.

Nutrition: Calories: 182, Fat: 5.1, Fiber: 3.4, Carbs: 12.3, Protein: 2.6

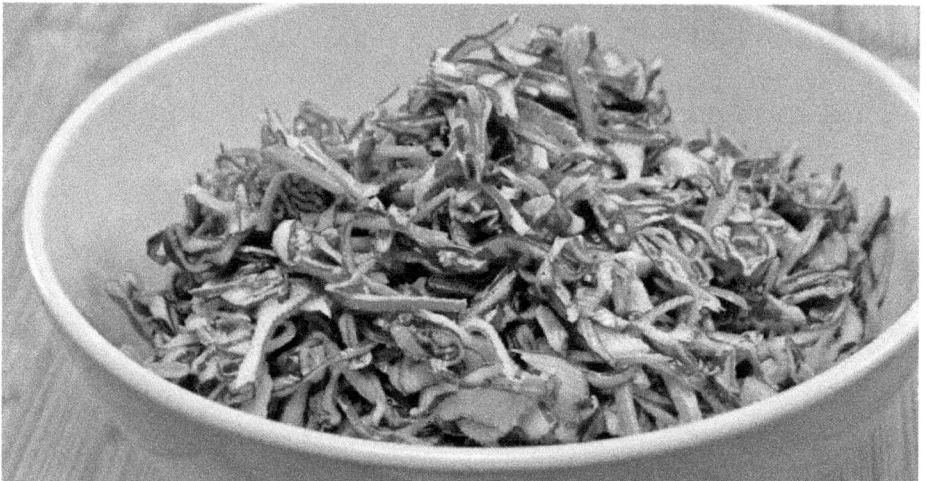

Spaghetti Squash and Leeks

Preparation Time: 15 minutes

Cooking Time: 10 minutes

Servings: 4

Ingredients:

2   leeks, sliced

1 teaspoon chili powder

1 teaspoon cumin, ground 1 teaspoon onion powder

1 teaspoon apple cider vinegar

1-pound spaghetti squash halved, seeds removed 1 tablespoon Italian seasoning

1   cup water for cooking

Directions:

1.   Add water and insert a steamer rack.

2.   Arrange spaghetti squash on the rack and close the lid.

3.   Cook it on High for 10 minutes. Then allow natural pressure release for 5 minutes.

4.   Check if the spaghetti squash is soft, shred the flesh with the help of a fork, and transfer it to a bowl.

5.   Toss and serve.

Nutrition: Calories: 110, Fat: 1.7, Fiber: 0, Carbs: 4.3, Protein: 0.8

Paprika Sweet Potato

Preparation Time: 10 minutes

Cooking Time: 11 minutes

Servings: 2

Ingredients:

2   sweet potatoes

2 teaspoons sweet paprika 1/2 teaspoon oregano, dried

1 teaspoon chili powder

1 teaspoon chives, chopped 1/2 cup of water

Directions:

1.   Add water and insert a steamer rack.

2.   Put potatoes on the rack and close the lid.

3.   Set Manual mode (High pressure) and cook for 11 minutes. Then use quick pressure release.

4.   Transfer the potatoes to the plate, cut into halves, sprinkle the rest of the ingredients on top, and serve.

Nutrition: Calories: 159, Fat: 3.4, Fiber: 2.8, Carbs: 33.8, Protein: 3.6

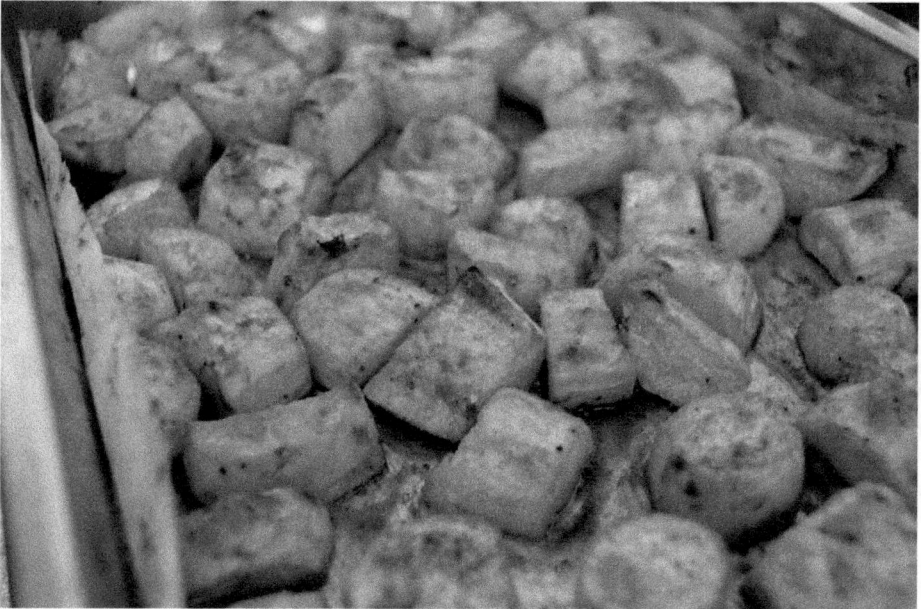

Cinnamon Carrots

Preparation Time: 10 minutes

Cooking Time: 15 minutes

Servings: 4

Ingredients:

1 pound baby carrots, scrubbed 1/3 cup water

1 tsp cinnamon

1/4 tsp chili powder

1 teaspoon black pepper

Directions:

1.   In the instant pot, mix the carrots with the water and the other ingredients, close the lid, and Manual mode (High pressure) for 15 minutes.

2.   After this, use quick pressure release.

3.   Divide between plates and serve.

Nutrition: Calories: 147, Fat: 0.5, Fiber: 7.1, Carbs: 9.9, Protein: 4.3

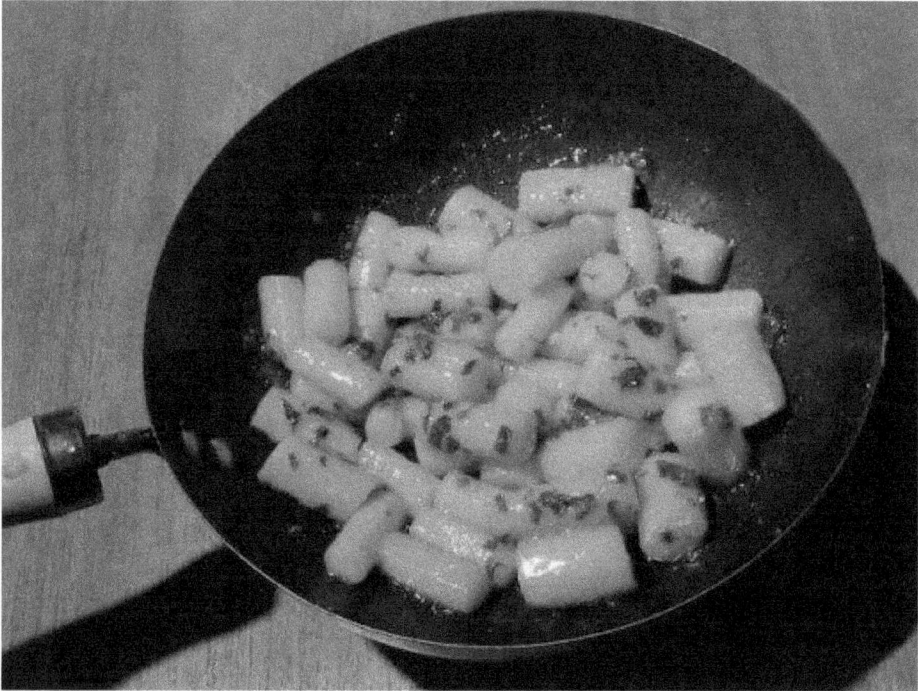

Wild Rice and Corn

Preparation Time: 10 minutes

Cooking Time: 8 minutes

Servings: 4

Ingredients:

1 cup wild rice

1 tablespoon Italian seasoning 1/4 cup corn kernels, canned 1 teaspoon chili powder

1   teaspoon salt

2   cups vegetable broth

1 tsp chives

2 tsp olive oil

Directions:

1.   Add oil and set Saute mode.

2.   Add rice and seasoning and cook for 2 minutes.

3.   Add the rest of the ingredients and toss.

4.   Set Manual mode (High pressure) and close the lid. Seal it.

5.   Cook rice for 6 minutes. Use quick pressure release.

Nutrition: Calories: 254 Fat: 4.3 Fiber: 1.5 Carbs: 25.4 Protein: 5.4

Jicama and Spinach Salad

Preparation Time: 10 minutes

Cooking Time: 20 minutes

Servings: 4

Ingredients:

Salad:

10 oz. baby spinach washed and dried Grape or cherry tomatoes, cut in half

1 jicama, washed, peeled, and cut in strips Green or Kalamata olives, chopped

8 tsp walnuts, chopped

1 tsp raw or roasted sunflower seeds Maple Mustard Dressing

Dressing:

1   heaping tbsp Dijon mustard Dash cayenne pepper

2   tbsp maple syrup

2 garlic cloves, minced 1 to 2 tbsp water

¼ tsp sea salt

Directions:

For the salad:

1.   Divide the baby spinach onto 4 salad plates. Top each serving with

¼ of the jicama, ¼ of the chopped olives, and 4 tomatoes. Sprinkle 1 tsp of the sunflower seeds and 2 tsp of the walnuts.

For the dressing:

2.   In a small mixing bowl, whisk all the ingredients together until emulsified. Check the taste and add more maple syrup for sweetness.

3.   Drizzle 1½ tbsp of the dressing over each salad and serve.

Nutrition:

Calories: 196 Fat: 2g Protein: 7g Carbs: 28g

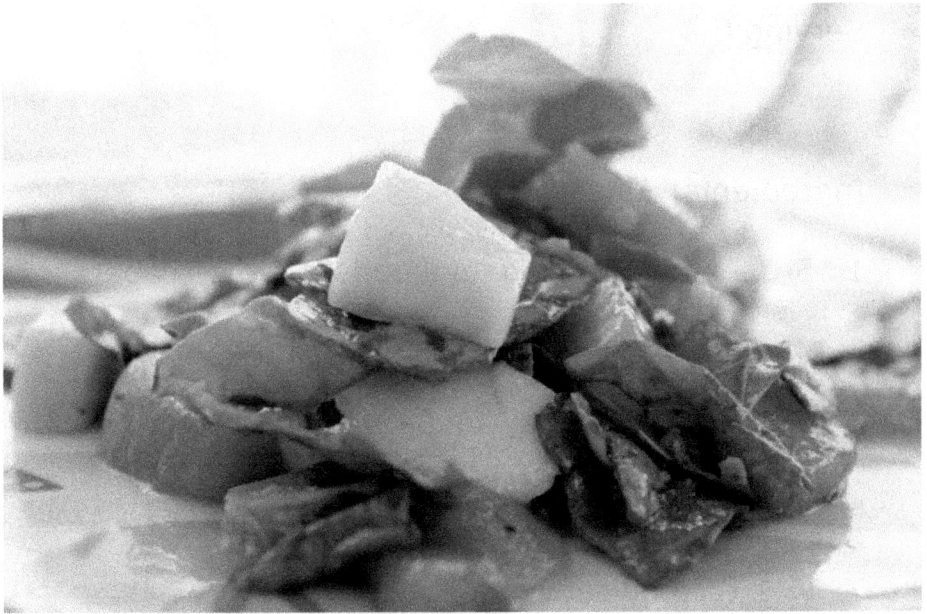

High-Protein Salad

Preparation Time: 5 minutes

Cooking Time: 5 minutes

Servings: 4

Ingredients: Salad:

1 15-oz. can green kidney beans 2 4 tbsp capers

3 4 handfuls arugula 4 15-oz. can lentils

5   1 tbsp caper brine

6   1 tbsp tamari

7   1 tbsp balsamic vinegar

8   2 tbsp peanut butter

9   2 tbsp hot sauce

10   1 tbsp tahini

Directions:

For the dressing:

1.   In a bowl, whisk together all the ingredients until they come together to form a smooth dressing.

For the salad:

2.   Mix the beans, arugula, capers, and lentils. Top with the dressing and serve.

Nutrition:

Calories: 205 Fat: 2g Protein: 13g Carbs: 31g

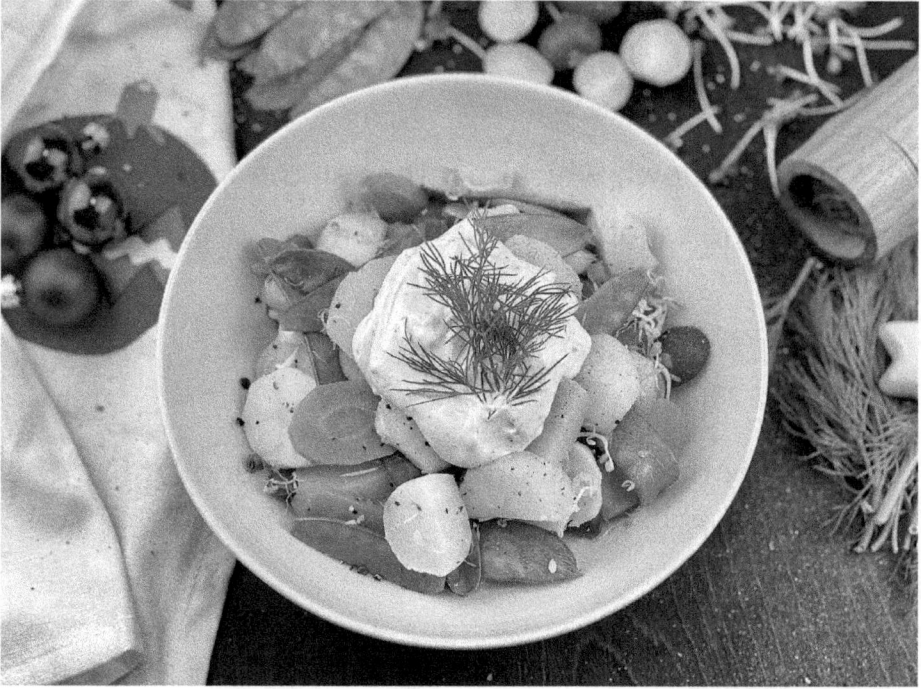

Southwest Style Salad

Preparation Time: 10 minutes

Cooking Time: 0 minutes

Servings: 3

Ingredients:

½ cup dry black beans

½ cup dry chickpeas

1/3 cup purple onion, diced

1 red bell pepper, pitted, sliced

4 cups mixed greens, fresh or frozen, chopped 1 cup cherry tomatoes, halved or quartered

1 medium avocado, peeled, pitted, and cubed 1 cup sweet kernel corn, canned, drained

½ tsp. chili powder

¼ tsp. cumin

¼ tsp Salt

¼ tsp pepper 2 tsp. olive oil

1 tbsp. vinegar

Directions:

1.	Prepare the black beans and chickpeas according to the method.

2.	Put all of the ingredients into a large bowl.

3.	Toss the mix of veggies and spices until combined thoroughly.

4.	Store, or serve chilled with some olive oil and vinegar on top!

Nutrition:

Calories: 635 Fat: 19.9g Carbs: 95.4g Protein: 24.3g

Shaved Brussel Sprout Salad

Preparation Time: 25 minutes

Cooking Time: 0 minutes

Servings: 4

Ingredients:

1   tbsp. brown mustard 1 tbsp. maple syrup

2   tbsp. apple cider vinegar 2 tbsp. extra virgin olive oil

½ tbsp. garlic minced

Dressing:

½ cup dry red kidney beans

¼ cup dry chickpeas

2 cups Brussel sprouts 1 cup purple onion

1 small sour apple

½ cup slivered almonds, crushed

½ cup walnuts, crushed

½ cup cranberries, dried

¼ tsp Salt

¼ tsp pepper

Directions:

1.   Prepare the beans according to the method.

2.   Combine all dressing ingredients in a bowl and stir well until combined.

3.   Refrigerate the dressing for up to one hour before serving.

4.   Using a greater mandolin or knife to slice each Brussel sprout thinly. Repeat this with the apple and onion.

5.   Take a large bowl to mix the chickpeas, beans, sprouts, apples, onions, cranberries, and nuts.

6.   Drizzle the cold dressing over the salad to coat.

7.   Serve with salt and pepper to taste, or store for later!

Nutrition:

Calories: 432 Fat: 23.5g Carbs: 45.3g Protein: 15.9g

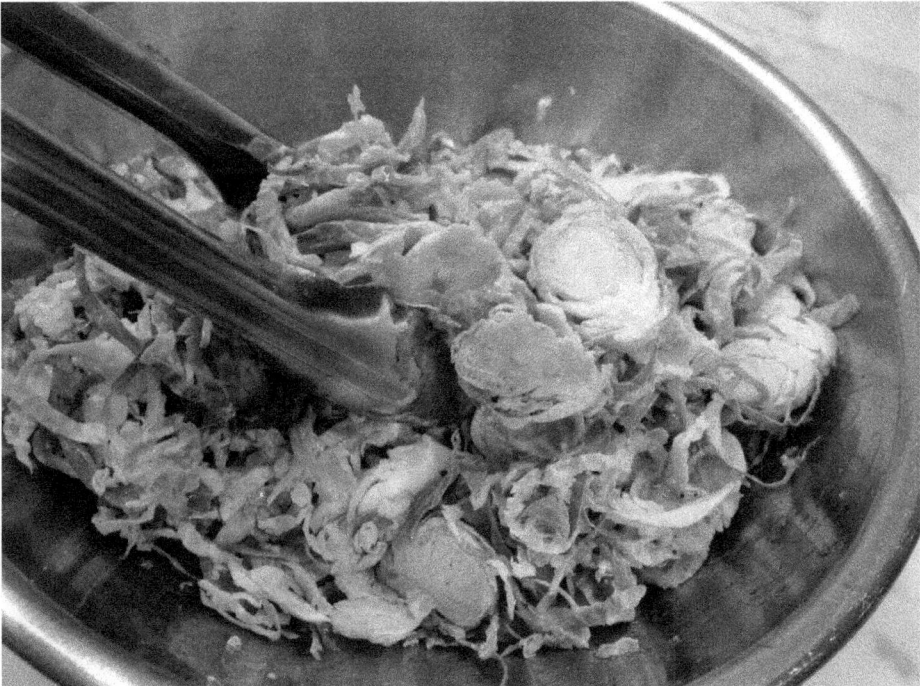

Colorful Protein Power Salad

Preparation Time: 20 minutes

Cooking Time: 0 minutes

Servings: 2

Ingredients:

½ cup dry quinoa

2   cups dry navy beans 1 green onion, chopped 2 tsp. garlic, minced

3   cups green or purple cabbage, chopped 4 cups kale, fresh or frozen, chopped

1 cup shredded carrot, chopped 2 tbsp. extra virgin olive oil

1 tsp. lemon juice

¼ tsp Salt

¼ tsp pepper

Directions:

1.   Prepare the quinoa according to the recipe.

2.   Prepare the beans according to the method.

3.   Put 1 tbsp of oil on a frying pan

4.   Add the chopped green onion, garlic, cabbage, and sauté for 2- 3 minutes.

5.   Add the kale, the remaining 1 tablespoon of olive oil, and salt. Lower the heat and cover until the greens have wilted, around 5 minutes. Remove the pan from the stove and set it aside.

6.   Take a large bowl and mix the remaining ingredients with the kale and cabbage mixture once it has cooled down. Add more salt and pepper to taste.

7.   Mix until everything is distributed evenly.

8.   Serve topped with a dressing, or store for later!

Nutrition:

Calories: 1100 Fat: 19.9g Carbs: 180.8g Protein: 58.6g

Lemon Cauliflower

Preparation Time: 7 minutes

Cooking Time: 8 minutes

Servings: 4

Ingredients:

1-pound cauliflower florets 1 teaspoon lemon zest

1 tablespoon lemon juice

1 tsp turmeric powder

1 tsp pepper

1 teaspoon Pink salt

1 tablespoon fresh dill, chopped 1/4 cup vegetable broth

1 tablespoon olive oil

Directions:

1.   In the instant pot, mix the cauliflower with the lemon juice, zest, and the other ingredients, close the lid and cook on Manual mode for 8 minutes.

2.   Allow natural pressure release.

Nutrition: Calories: 205, Fat: 4.5g, Fiber: 3.3g, Carbs: 14.5g, Protein: 4.2g

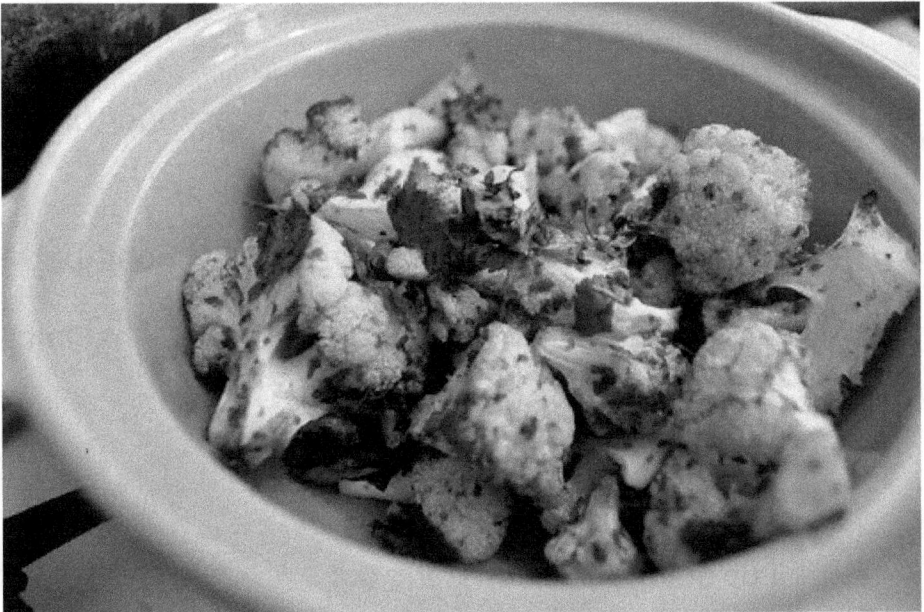

Lemongrass Rice

Preparation Time: 15 minutes

Cooking Time: 15 minutes

Servings: .3

Ingredients:

1 cup wild rice

1 cup vegetable broth

1 tablespoon lemongrass, chopped 1 teaspoon turmeric powder

1 teaspoon oregano, dried 1 tablespoon almond butter

3/4 teaspoon ground nutmeg 1/3 teaspoon Pink salt

Directions:

1.   Put quinoa in an instant pot.

2.   Add the remainings ingredients and toss. Close the lid, seal it, and set Manual mode (high pressure).

3.   Cook for 15 minutes and allow natural pressure release for 10 minutes.

4.   Divide between plates and serve.

Nutrition: Calories: 225, Fat: 7.1g, Fiber: 4.6g, Carbs: 22.3g, Protein: 10.8g

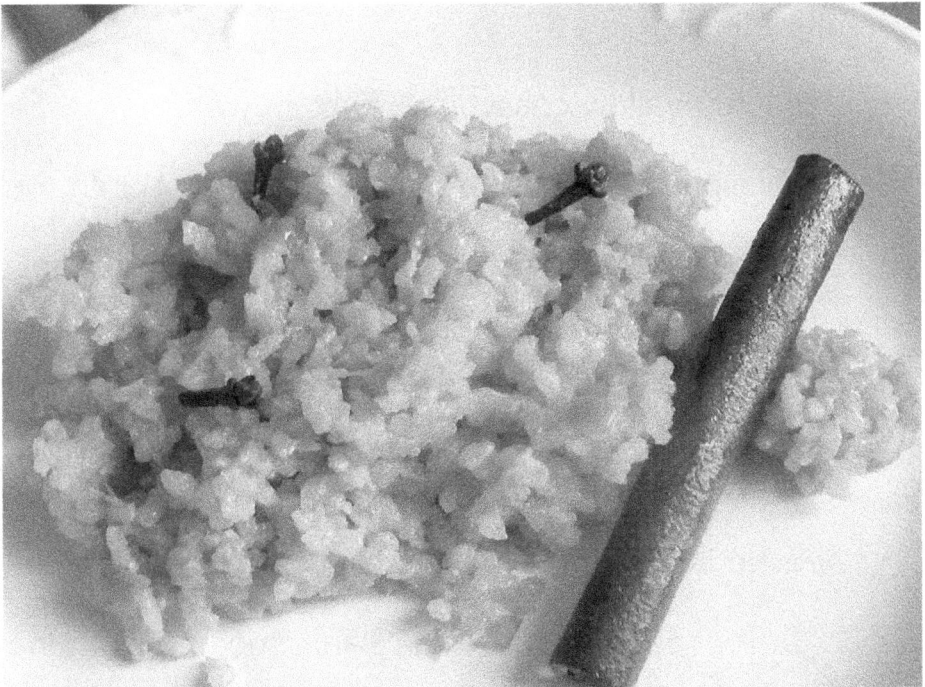

Chives Couscous

Preparation Time: 15 minutes

Cooking Time: 5 minutes

Servings: 4

Ingredients:

1 1/2 cup yellow couscous 2 cups of water

1 tablespoon chives, chopped 1 teaspoon cumin, ground

1 teaspoon coriander, ground 1 teaspoon cayenne pepper

1 tablespoon olive oil 1 teaspoon salt

Directions:

1.   Preheat instant pot on Saute mode for 3 minutes.

2.   Pour olive oil inside it and add couscous.

3.   Stir it gently and saute for 2 minutes.

4.   Add the remaining ingredients and toss. Close the lid. Set manual mode (High pressure).

5.   Cook the side dish for 2 minutes.

6.   Release the pressure manually for 10 minutes.

Nutrition: Calories: 96, Fat: 3.6g, Fiber: 0.8g, Carbs: 11.5g, Protein: 4.5g

Coconut Cauliflower Mix

Preparation Time: 10 minutes

Cooking Time: 10 minutes

Servings: 6

Ingredients:

1-pound cauliflower florets 1 cup of water

1/4 cup of coconut milk

1 tablespoon coconut yogurt 1 teaspoon salt

1 teaspoon hot paprika

1 teaspoon Italian seasoning 1 tablespoon chives, chopped

Directions:

1.   Place cauliflower and water in the instant pot. Add salt and close the lid.

2.   Cook the vegetables on Manual mode for 10 minutes.

3.   Then use quick pressure release.

4.   Open the lid, drain water and mash the cauliflower.

5.   Add the remainings ingredients, stir well and serve.

Nutrition: Calories: 211, Fat: 4.6g, Fiber: 5.3g, Carbs: 24.2g, Protein: 3.9g

Peppers Bowl

Preparation Time: 10 minutes

Cooking Time: 10 minutes

Servings: 2

Ingredients:

1-pound red bell peppers, roughly sliced 1/2 red onion, chopped

1 tsp salt

1 tsp pepper 1 teaspoon chili powder

1/2 jalapeno pepper, chopped 1/2 cup vegetable stock

1/4 teaspoon ground coriander 1 teaspoon dried rosemary

1   teaspoon olive oil

Directions:

1.   In the instant pot, mix the peppers with the onion, salt, and the other ingredients except for the

stock, set the pot on Saute mode, and saute for 3 minutes.

2.   Then the stock. Close the lid and set manual mode (High pressure) for 7 minutes.

3.   Make a quick pressure release.

4.   Transfer into the bowls.

Nutrition: Calories: 201g, Fat: 4.3g, Fiber: 3.8g, Carbs: 14.3g, Protein: 5.3g

Chili Cauliflower Rice

Preparation Time: 10 minutes

Cooking Time: 6 minutes

Servings: 4

Ingredients:

2   1/2 cup cauliflower florets, grated 1 teaspoon black pepper

1 teaspoon oregano, dried

1 teaspoon turmeric powder 1 teaspoon salt

1/2 cup of water

1 teaspoon olive oil

1 tablespoon chives, chopped

Directions:

1.   In an instant pot, mix the cauliflower rice with black pepper and the other ingredients and close the lid.

2.   Set manual mode and cook on High for 6 minutes. Make a quick pressure release.

3.   Chill the cauliflower rice for 2-5 minutes before serving.

Nutrition: Calories: 32, Fat: 1.4g, Fiber: 1.6g, Carbs: 3.5g, Protein: 1.7g

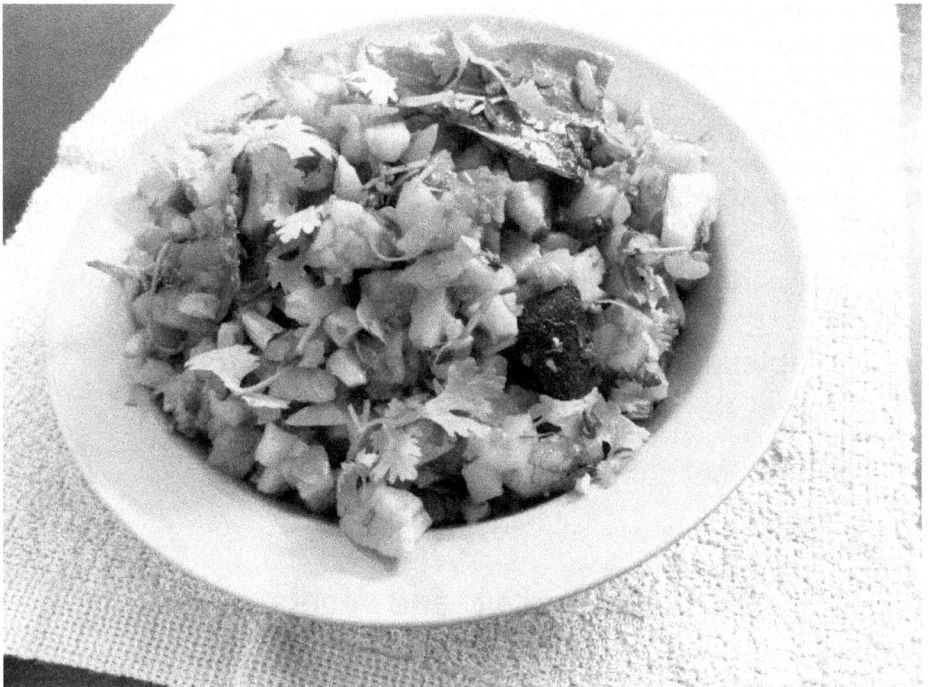

Potato Mash

Preparation Time: 10 minutes

Cooking Time: 9 minutes

Servings: 6

Ingredients:

1 and 1/2 lb.' white potatoes, peeled, chopped 1 teaspoon salt

1/2 teaspoon hot paprika 1 teaspoon dill, dried

1 tablespoon coconut butter

1 teaspoon ground black pepper 1 cup vegetable broth

1 tablespoon fresh parsley, chopped

Directions:

1.   Put potatoes, salt, and vegetable broth in the instant pot.

2.   Close the lid and set manual mode. Cook on High for 9 minutes.

3. Then make quick pressure release, strain the sweet potatoes and mash until smooth.

4. Add the remainings ingredients, stir well and serve.

Nutrition: Calories: 123, Fat: 4.3g, Fiber: 2.2g, Carbs: 11.4g, Protein: 4.3g

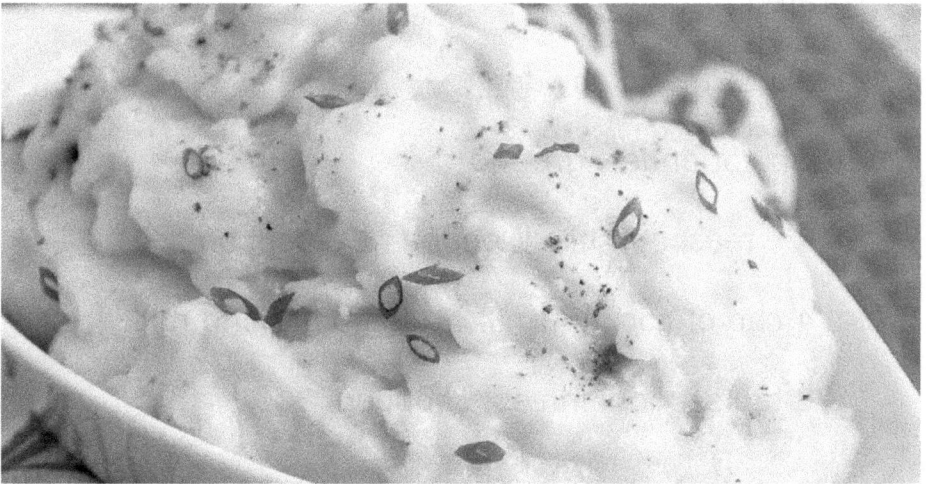

Red Cabbage and Carrots

Preparation Time: 10 minutes

Cooking Time: 7 minutes

Servings: 3

Ingredients:

1-pound red cabbage, shredded 2 carrots, peeled and grated

1 tsp turmeric powder

1 tsp coriander, ground

1   teaspoon black pepper 1 teaspoon salt

1/4 cup of coconut milk 3/4 cup almond milk

1/2 tablespoon chives, chopped

Directions:

1.   In an instant pot, mix the cabbage with the carrots and the other ingredients, toss and set manual mode (High pressure).

2.   Cook the cabbage for 7 minutes. Then allow natural pressure release.

3.   Transfer the meal into the serving bowls and cool down before serving.

Nutrition: Calories: 182, Fat: 5.1g, Fiber: 3.4g, Carbs: 12.3g, Protein: 2.6g

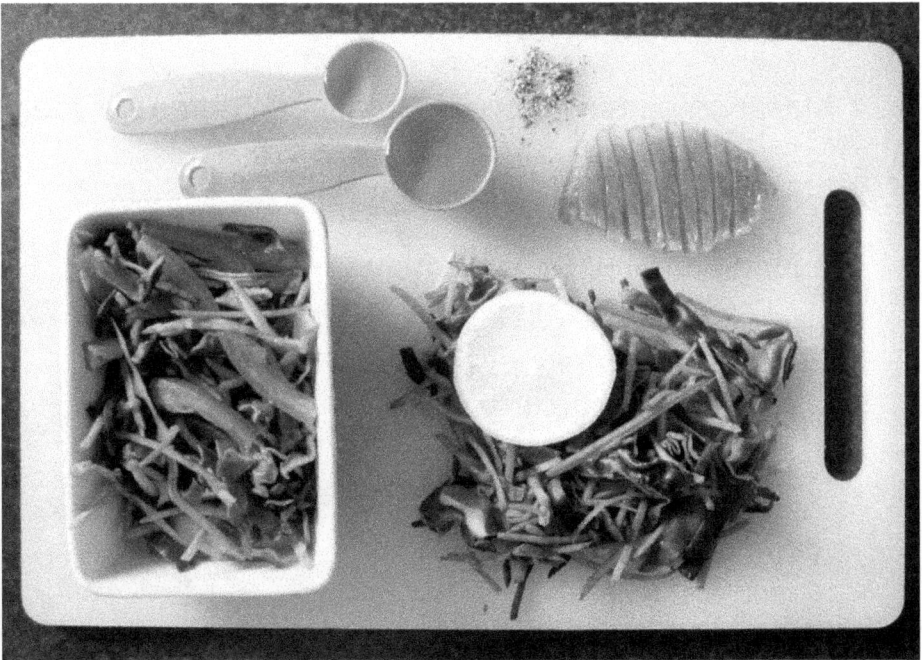

Spaghetti Squash and Leeks

Preparation Time: 15 minutes

Cooking Time: 10 minutes

Servings: 4

Ingredients:

2   leeks, sliced

1 teaspoon chili powder

1 teaspoon cumin, ground 1 teaspoon onion powder

1 teaspoon apple cider vinegar

1-pound spaghetti squash halved, seeds removed 1 tablespoon Italian seasoning

1 cup water for cooking

Directions:

1.   Put water into a steamer rack.

2.   Arrange spaghetti squash on the rack and close the lid.

3.	Cook it on High for 10 minutes. Then allow natural pressure release for 5 minutes.

4.	Check if the spaghetti squash is soft, shred the flesh with a fork's help, and transfer it to a bowl.

5.	Add the remainings ingredients, toss and serve.

Nutrition: Calories: 110, Fat: 1.7g, Fiber: 9g, Carbs: 4.3g, Protein: 2.8g

Paprika Sweet Potato

Preparation Time: 10 minutes

Cooking Time: 11 minutes

Servings: 2

Ingredients:

2   sweet potatoes

2 teaspoons sweet paprika 1/2 teaspoon oregano, dried
1 teaspoon chili powder

1 teaspoon chives, chopped 1/2 cup of water

Directions:

1.   Add water and put in a steamer rack.

2.   Put potatoes on the rack and close the lid.

3.   Set Manual mode (High pressure) and cook for 11 minutes. Then use quick pressure release.

4.   Transfer the potatoes to the plate, cut into halves, sprinkle the rest of the ingredients on top, and serve.

Nutrition: Calories: 159, Fat: 3.4g, Fiber: 2.8g, Carbs: 33.8g, Protein: 3.6g

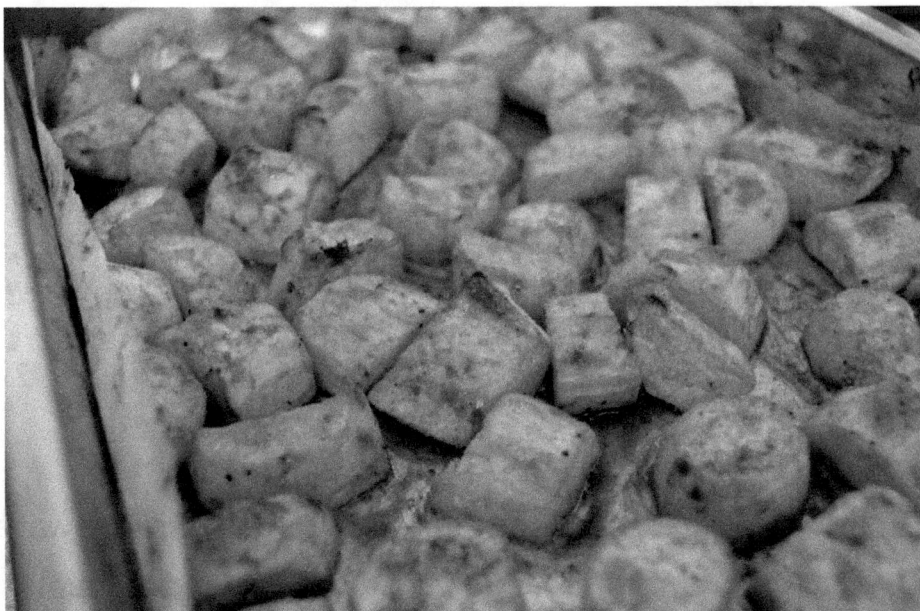

Cinnamon Carrots

Preparation Time: 10 minutes

Cooking Time: 15 minutes

Servings: 4

Ingredients:

1-pound baby carrots scrubbed 1/3 cup water

1 tsp cinnamon

1/4 tsp chili powder

1 teaspoon black pepper

Directions:

1.   In the instant pot, mix the carrots with the water and the other ingredients, close the lid, and Manual mode (High pressure) for 15 minutes.

2.   After this, use quick pressure release.

3.   Divide between plates and serve.

Nutrition: Calories: 147, Fat: 0.5g, Fiber: 7.1g, Carbs: 9.9g, Protein: 4.3g

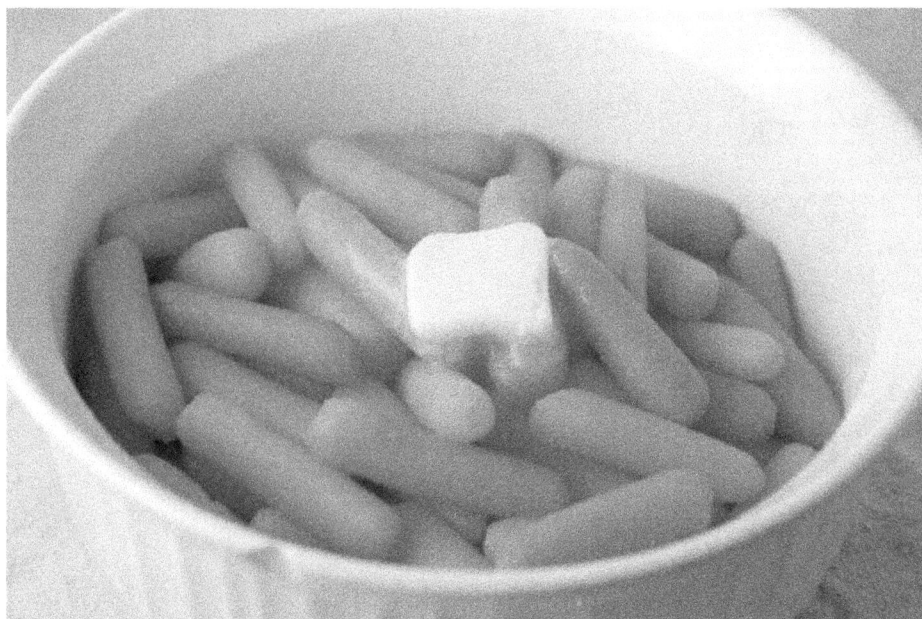

Potato Tuna Salad

Preparation Time: 4 hours and 20 minutes

Cooking Time: 10 minutes

Servings: 6

Ingredients:

Water

3 potatoes, peeled and sliced into cubes

½ cup plain yogurt

½ cup mayonnaise

1 garlic

1 tablespoon almond milk

1 tablespoon fresh dill, chopped

½ teaspoon lemon zest Salt to taste

1   cup cucumber, chopped

¼ cup scallions, chopped

¼ cup radishes, chopped 9 oz. canned tuna flakes

2   hard-boiled eggs, chopped 6 cups lettuce, chopped

Instructions:

1.   Fill your pot with water. Add the potatoes and oil.

2.   Cook for 8 minutes.

3.   Drain and let cool.

4.   In a bowl, mix the yogurt, mayo, garlic, almond milk, fresh dill, lemon zest, and salt.

5.   Stir in the potatoes, tuna flakes, and eggs. Mix well.

6.   Chill in the refrigerator for 4 hours.

7.   Stir in the shredded lettuce before serving.

Nutrition: Calories: 243 Fat: 9.9g Carbs: 22.2g Protein: 17.5g

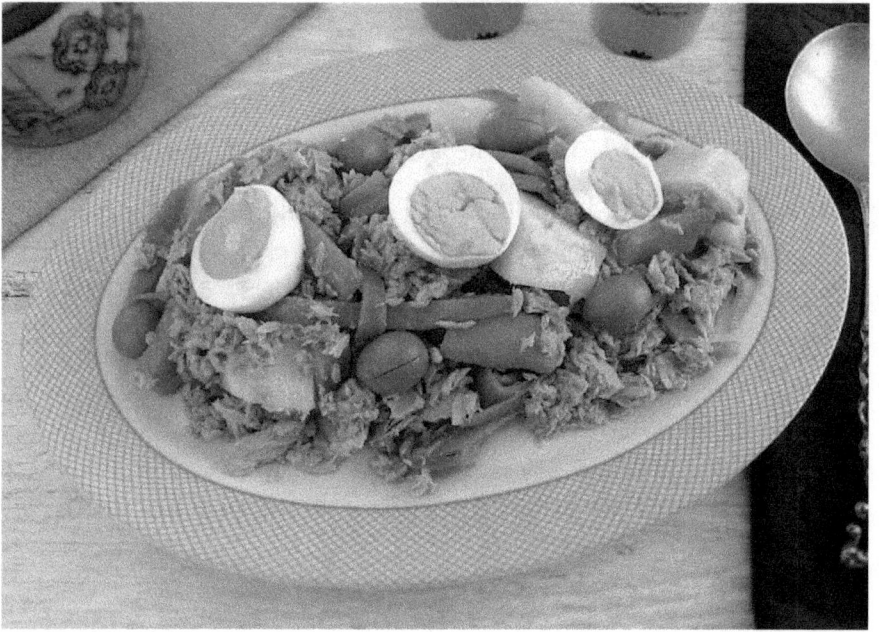

Shrimp Veggie Pasta Salad

Preparation Time: 50 minutes

Cooking Time: 10 minutes

Servings: 6

Ingredients:

1 lb. shrimp, peeled and deveined 8 oz. asparagus, sliced

Salt and pepper to taste

12 oz. farfalle, penne or macaroni pasta, cooked 2 tablespoons parsley, chopped

½ cup shallots, sliced thinly

¼ cup Parmesan cheese, grated

2 tablespoons freshly squeezed lemon juice

½ cup mayonnaise

2 teaspoons garlic, minced

1 teaspoon Worcestershire sauce 1 teaspoon Dijon mustard

1 lemon, sliced into wedges

Instructions:

1.   Preheat your oven to 400°F.

2.   Arrange the shrimp and asparagus in a baking pan.

3.   Season with salt and pepper.

4.   Roast in the oven for 10 minutes.

5.   Let cool. Transfer to a bowl.

6.   Stir in the cooked pasta, parsley, and shallots.

7.   Sprinkle the Parmesan cheese on top.

8.   In another bowl, combine the lemon juice, mayonnaise, garlic, Worcestershire sauce, and Dijon mustard.

9.   Add this mixture to the pasta salad. Toss to coat evenly.

10.   Put into fridge for 28 minutes before serving.

11.   Garnish with lemon wedges.

Nutrition:

Calories: 429

Fat: 17.1g Carbs: 45.6g Protein: 25g

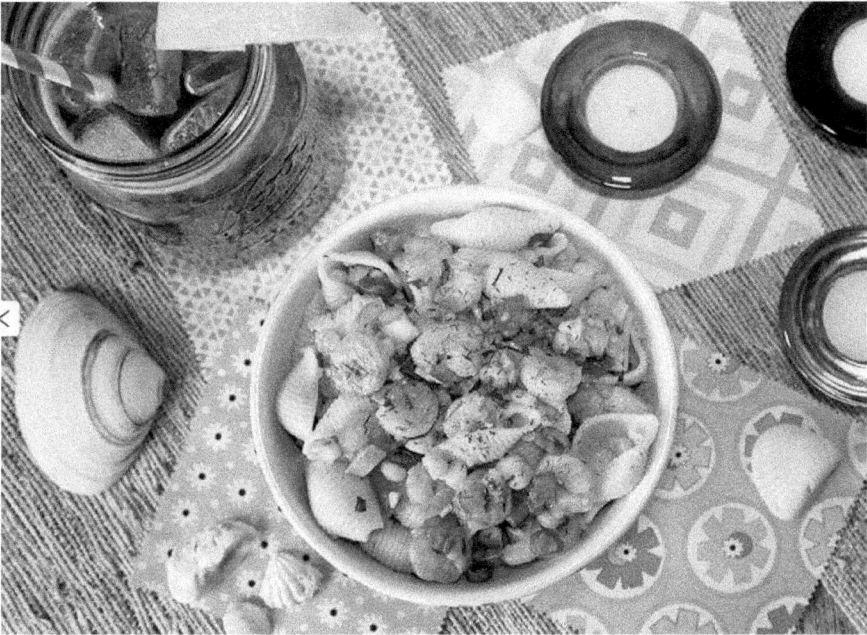

Coconut Cauliflower Mix

Preparation Time: 10 minutes

Cooking Time: 10 minutes

Servings: 6

Ingredients:

1 pound cauliflower florets 1 cup of water

1/4 cup of coconut milk

1 tablespoon coconut yogurt 1 teaspoon salt

1 teaspoon hot paprika

1 teaspoon Italian seasoning 1 tablespoon chives, chopped

Directions:

1.   Place cauliflower and water in the instant pot. Add salt and close the lid.

2.   Cook the vegetables on Manual mode for 10 minutes.

3.   Then use quick pressure release.

4.   Open the lid, drain water and mash the cauliflower.

5.   Stir well and serve.

Nutrition: Calories: 211, Fat: 4.6, Fiber: 5.3, Carbs: 24.2, Protein: 3.9

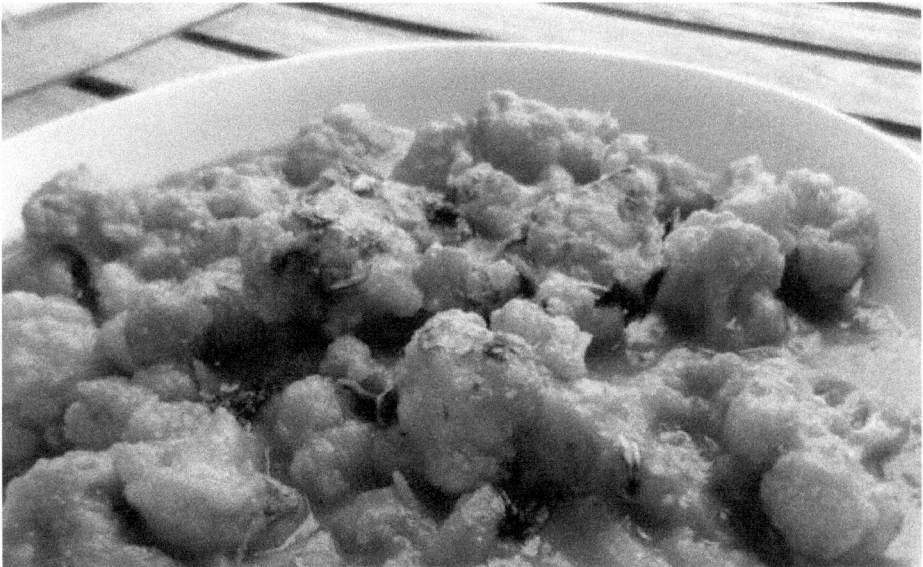

Peppers Bowl

Preparation Time: 10 minutes

Cooking Time: 10 minutes

Servings: 2

Ingredients:

1 pound red bell peppers, roughly sliced 1/2 red onion, chopped

1 tsp salt

1 tsp pepper

1 tsp chili powder

1/2 jalapeno pepper, chopped 1/2 cup vegetable stock

1/4 teaspoon ground coriander 1 teaspoon dried rosemary

1   teaspoon olive oil

Directions:

1.   In the instant pot, mix the peppers with the onion, salt, and the other ingredients except for the stock, set the pot on Saute mode, and saute for 3 minutes.

2.   Then the stock. Close the lid and set manual mode (High pressure) for 7 minutes.

3.   Make a quick pressure release.

4.   Transfer into the bowls.

Nutrition: Calories: 201, Fat: 4.3, Fiber: 3.8, Carbs: 14.3, Protein: 5.3

Chili Cauliflower Rice

Preparation Time: 10 minutes

Cooking Time: 6 minutes

Servings: 4

Ingredients:

2   1/2 cup cauliflower florets, grated 1 teaspoon black pepper

1 teaspoon oregano, dried

1 teaspoon turmeric powder 1 teaspoon salt

1/2 cup of water

1 teaspoon olive oil

1 tablespoon chives, chopped

Directions:

1.   In the instant pot, mix the cauliflower rice with black pepper and the other ingredients and close the lid.

2.   Set manual mode and cook on High for 6 minutes. Make a quick pressure release.

3.   Chill the cauliflower rice for 2-5 minutes before serving.

Nutrition: Calories: 32, Fat: 1.4, Fiber: 1.6, Carbs: 3.5, Protein: 1.7

Edamame & Ginger Citrus Salad

Preparation Time: 15 minutes

Cooking Time: 0 minutes

Servings: 3

Ingredients:

¼ cup orange juice 1 tsp. lime juice

½ tbsp. maple syrup

½ tsp. ginger, finely minced

½ tbsp. sesame oil

Dressing:

 ½ cup dry green lentils 2 cups carrots, shredded

4   cups kale, fresh or frozen, chopped 1 cup edamame, shelled

1 tablespoon roasted sesame seeds 2 tsp. mint, chopped

Salt and pepper to taste

1 small avocado, peeled, pitted, diced

Directions:

1.   Prepare the lentils according to the method.

2.   Combine the orange and lime juices, maple syrup, and ginger in a small bowl. Mix with a whisk while slowly adding the sesame oil.

3.   Add the cooked lentils, carrots, kale, edamame, sesame seeds, and mint to a large bowl.

4.   Add the dressing and stir well until all the ingredients are coated evenly.

5.   Store or serve topped with avocado and an additional sprinkle of mint.

Nutrition:

Calories: 507 Fat: 23.1g Carbs: 56.8g Protein: 24.6g

Taco Tempeh Salad

Preparation Time: 25 minutes

Cooking Time: 0 minutes

Servings: 3

Ingredients:

1 cup dry black beans

1 8-oz. package tempeh

1 tbsp. lime or lemon juice 2 tbsp. extra virgin olive oil
1 tsp. maple syrup

½ tsp. chili powder

¼ tsp. cumin

¼ tsp. paprika

1 large bunch of kale, fresh or frozen, chopped 1 large avocado, peeled, pitted, diced

½ cup salsa

¼ tsp Salt

¼ tsp pepper

Directions:

1.   Prepare the beans according to the method.

2.   Cut the tempeh into ¼-inch cubes, place in a bowl, and then add the lime or lemon juice, 1 tablespoon of olive oil, maple syrup, chili powder, cumin, and paprika.

3.   Stir well and let the tempeh marinate in the fridge for at least 1 hour, up to 12 hours.

4.   Heat the remaining 1 tablespoon of olive oil in a frying pan over medium heat.

5.   Add the marinated tempeh mixture and cook until brown and crispy on both sides, around 10 minutes.

6.   Put the chopped kale in a bowl with the cooked beans and prepared tempeh.

7.   Store or serve the salad immediately, topped with salsa, avocado, and salt and pepper to taste.

Nutrition:

Calories: 627 Fat: 31.7g Carbs: 62.7g Protein: 31.4g

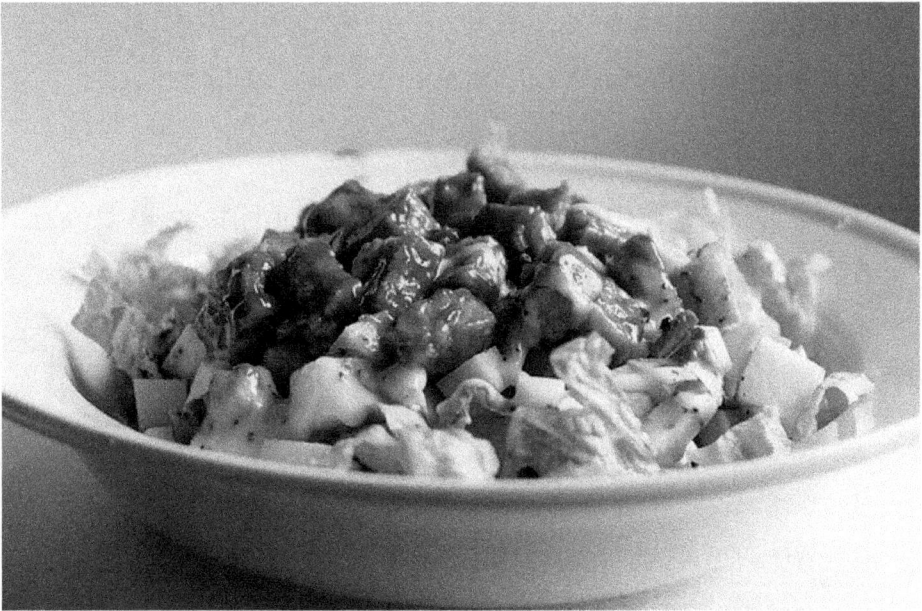

Lebanese Potato Salad

Preparation Time: 5 minutes

Cooking Time: 10 minutes

Servings: 4

Ingredients:

1-pound Russet potatoes

1   ½ tablespoon e.v.o. oil

2 scallions

Freshly ground pepper to taste 2 tablespoons lemon juice

¼ teaspoon salt or to taste

2   tablespoons fresh mint leaves, chopped

Directions:

1. Place a saucepan half-filled with water over medium heat. Add salt and potatoes and cook for 10 minutes until tender. Place potatoesin a bowl of cold water. When cool enough to handle, peel and cube the potatoes. Place in a bowl.

To make the dressing:

2. Add oil, lemon juice, salt, and pepper in a bowl and whisk well. Drizzle dressing over the potatoes. Toss well.

3. Add scallions and mint and toss well.

4. Divide into 4 plates and serve.

Nutrition:

Calories: 129 Fat: 5.5g Carbs: 18.8g Protein: 2.2g

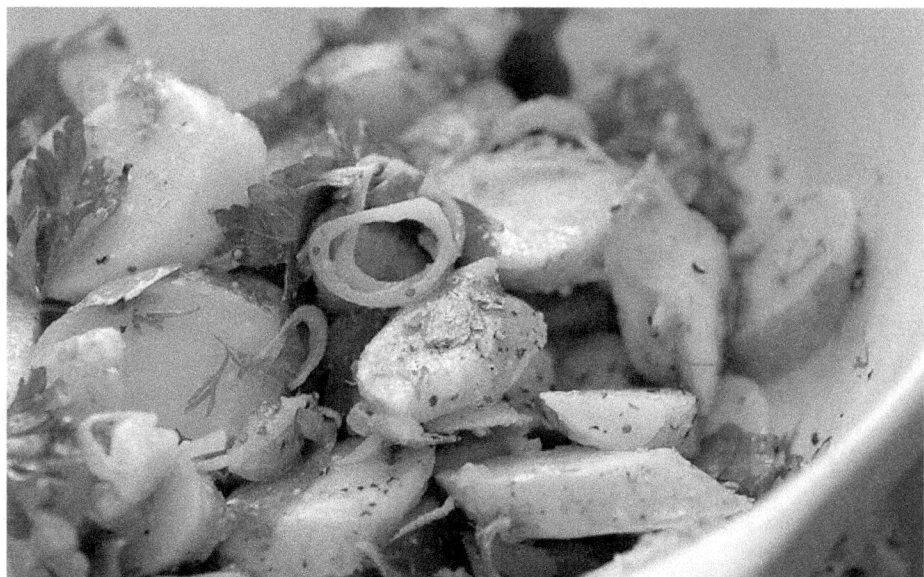

Chickpea and Spinach Salad

Preparation Time: 5 minutes

Cooking Time: 0 minutes

Servings: 4

Ingredients:

2 cans (14.5 oz. each) chickpeas, drained, rinsed 7 oz. vegan feta cheese, crumbled or chopped

1   tablespoon lemon juice 1/3 -½ cup olive oil

½ teaspoon salt or to taste 4-6 cups spinach, torn

½ cup raisins

2   tablespoons honey

1-2 teaspoons ground cumin 1 teaspoon chili flakes

Directions:

1.   Add cheese, chickpeas, and spinach into a large bowl.

2.   Make the dressing: Add the rest of the ingredients into another bowl and mix well.

3.   Pour dressing over the salad. Toss well and serve.

Nutrition:

Calories: 822 Fat: 42.5g Carbs: 89.6g Protein: 29g

Wild Rice and Corn

Preparation Time: 10 minutes

Cooking Time: 8 minutes

Servings: 4

Ingredients:

1 cup wild rice

1 tablespoon Italian seasoning 1/4 cup corn kernels, canned 1 teaspoon chili powder

1   teaspoon salt

2   cups vegetable broth

1 tsp chives

2 tsp olive oil

Directions:

1.   Saute olive

2.   Add rice and seasoning and cook for 2 minutes.

3.   Add the rest of the ingredients and toss.

4.   Set Manual mode (High pressure) and close the lid. Seal it.

5.   Cook rice for 6 minutes. Use quick pressure release.

Nutrition: Calories: 254, Fat: 4.3g, Carbs: 25.4, Protein: 5.4g

Kale Polenta

Preparation Time: 5 minutes

Cooking Time: 8 minutes

Servings: 5

Ingredients:

1 cup polenta

1/2 cup kale, chopped

1   tsp turmeric powder

1 tsp smoked paprika

4 cups vegetable broth

2   tablespoons coconut milk

1/2 tsp pepper

1 teaspoon salt

Directions:

1.   Whisk together polenta and vegetable broth.

2.   Pour mixture into the instant pot, add the rest of the ingredients and toss.

3.   Close the lid and cook it on Manual mode (High pressure) for 8 minutes. Use quick pressure release/

4.   Transfer cooked polenta to the bowl, stir and serve.

Nutrition: Calories: 182, Fat: 2.8g, Fiber: 1g, Carbs: 20.5g, Protein: 6.3g

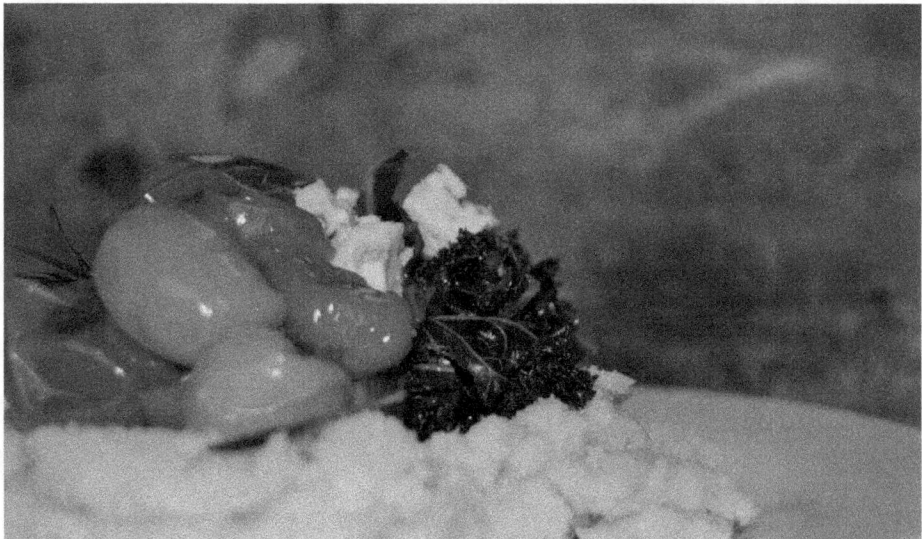

Broccoli Salad

Preparation Time: 5 minutes

Cooking Time: 25 minutes

Servings: 6

Ingredients:

2 tablespoons sherry vinegar

¼ cup olive oil

2 tsp thyme

1 tsp Dijon mustard

1 teaspoon honey Salt to taste

8 cups broccoli florets, steamed or roasted 2 red onions, sliced thinly

½ cup Parmesan cheese shaved

¼ cup pecans, toasted and chopped

Directions:

1.   Mix the sherry vinegar, olive oil, thyme, mustard, honey, and salt in a bowl.

2.   In a serving bowl, combine the broccoli florets and onions.

3.   Drizzle the dressing on top.

4.   Sprinkle with the pecans and Parmesan cheese before serving.

Nutrition:

Calories: 199 Fat: 17.4g Carbs: 7.5g Protein: 5.2g

Potato Carrot Salad

Preparation Time: 15 minutes

Cooking Time: 10 minutes

Servings: 6

Ingredients:

Water

6 potatoes, sliced into cubes 3 carrots, sliced into cubes 1 tablespoon milk

1   tablespoon Dijon mustard

¼ cup mayonnaise Pepper to taste

2   teaspoons fresh thyme, chopped 1 stalk celery, chopped

2 scallions, chopped

1 slice turkey bacon, cooked crispy and crumbled

Directions:

1.   Fill your pot with water.

2.   Place it over medium-high heat.

3.   Boil the potatoes and carrots for 10 minutes or until tender.

4.   Drain and let cool.

5.   In a bowl, mix the milk mustard, mayo, pepper, and thyme.

6.   Stir in the potatoes, carrots, and celery.

7.   Coat evenly with the sauce.

8.   Cover and refrigerate for 4 hours.

9.   Top with the scallions and turkey bacon bits before serving.

Nutrition:

Calories: 106

Fat: 5.3

Carbs: 12.6g Protein: 2g

Penne with Veggies

Preparation Time: 5 minutes

Cooking Time: 25 minutes

Servings: 6

Ingredients:

2 teaspoons olive oil

2 cloves garlic, crushed and minced

½ cup shallots, chopped

2 tablespoons dry white wine

1 cup Brussels sprouts, trimmed and chopped 6 cups bok choy, chopped

6 cups cooked penne pasta

1   tablespoon vegetable oil spread Salt and pepper to taste

2   teaspoons dried Italian seasoning

3   tablespoons Parmesan cheese, grated

Directions:

2.   Put oil in a pan.

3.   Cook the garlic for 3 minutes.

4.   Pour in the wine.

5.   Scrape the browned bits using a wooden spoon.

6.   Stir in the Brussels sprouts.

7.   Cook for 3 minutes.

8.   Stir in the bok choy and cook for 2 to 3 minutes.

9.   Toss the pasta in the veggies.

10.   Add the vegetable oil into the mix.

11.   Season with salt, pepper, and Italian seasoning.

12.   Sprinkle the Parmesan cheese on top.

Nutrition:

Calories: 27 Fat: 4g Carbs: 17g Protein: 6g

Marinated Veggie Salad

Preparation Time: 4 hours and 30 minutes

Cooking Time:

Servings: 6

Ingredients:

1 zucchini, sliced

4 tomatoes, sliced into wedges

¼ cup red onion, sliced thinly 1 green bell pepper, sliced

2 tablespoons fresh parsley, chopped 2 tablespoons red-wine vinegar

2 tbsp olive oil

1 clove garlic

1 teaspoon dried basil 2 tablespoons water

Pine nuts, toasted and chopped

Instructions:

1. In a bowl, combine the zucchini, tomatoes, red onion, green bell pepper, and parsley.

2. Pour the vinegar and oil into a glass jar with a lid.

3. Add the garlic, basil, and water.

4. Seal the jar and shake well to combine.

5. Pour the dressing into the vegetable mixture.

6. Cover the bowl.

7. Marinate in the refrigerator for 4 hours.

8. Garnish with the pine nuts before serving.

Nutrition: Calories: 65 Fat: 4.7g

Carbs: 5.3g Protein: 0.9g

Arugula Salad

Preparation Time: 15 minutes

Cooking Time: 0 minute

Servings: 4

Ingredients:

6 cups fresh arugula leaves 2 cups radicchio, chopped

¼ cup low-Fat: balsamic vinaigrette

¼ cup pine nuts, toasted and chopped

Instructions:

1.   Arrange the arugula leaves in a serving bowl. Sprinkle the radicchio on top.

2.   Drizzle with the vinaigrette. Sprinkle the pine nuts on top.

Nutrition:

Calories: 85 Fat: 6.6g Carbs: 5.1g Protein: 2.2g

Mediterranean Salad

Preparation Time: 20 minutes

Cooking Time: 5 minutes

Servings: 2

Ingredients:

2 teaspoons balsamic vinegar 1 tablespoon basil pesto

1 cup lettuce

¼ cup broccoli florets, chopped

½ cup zucchini, chopped

¼ cup tomato, chopped

¼ cup yellow bell pepper, chopped 2 tablespoons feta cheese, crumbled

Instructions:

1.   Arrange the lettuce on a serving platter.

2.   Top with broccoli, zucchini, tomato, and bell pepper.

3.   In a bowl, mix the vinegar and pesto.

4.   Drizzle the dressing on top.

5.   Sprinkle the feta cheese and serve.

Nutrition:

Calories: 100 Fat: 6g Carbs: 7g Protein: 4g

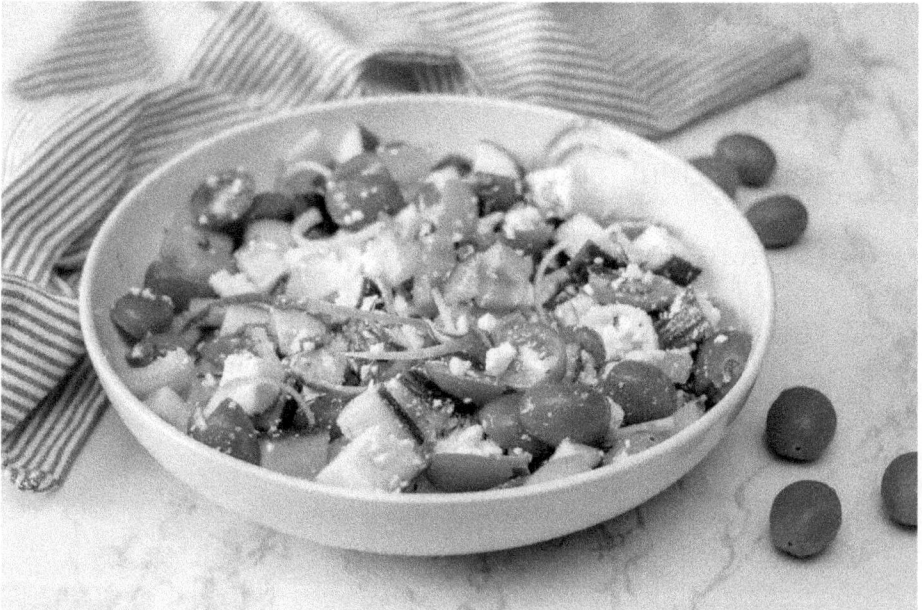

Tempeh "Chicken" Salad

Preparation Time: 10 minutes

Cooking Time: 0 minutes

Servings: 2

Ingredients:

4 tablespoons light mayonnaise 2 scallions, sliced

Pepper to taste

4 cups mixed salad greens 4 teaspoons white miso

2 tablespoons chopped fresh dill 1 ½ cups crumbled tempeh

1 cup sliced grape tomatoes

Directions:

To make the dressing:

1.   Add mayonnaise, scallions, miso, dill, and pepper into a bowl and whisk well.

2.   Add tempeh and fold gently. To serve:

3.   Divide the greens into 4 plates. Divide the tempeh among the plates. Top with tomatoes and serve.

Nutrition:

Calories: 452 Fat: 24.5g Carbs: 37.2g Protein: 29.9g

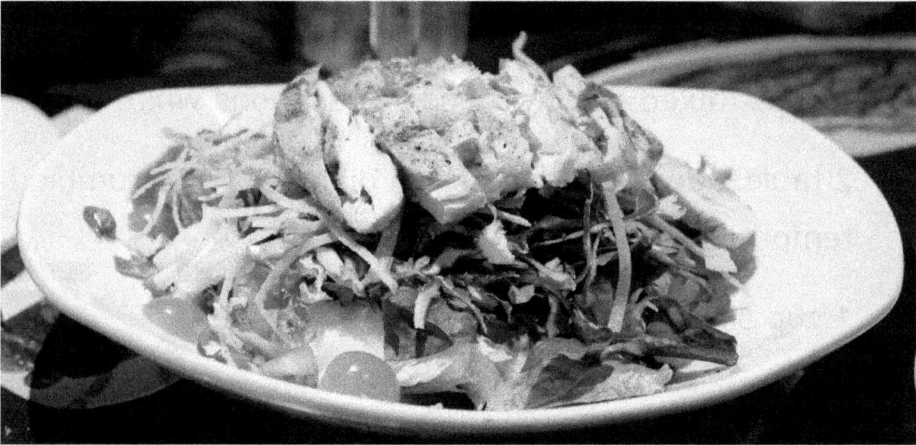

Spinach & Dill Pasta Salad

Preparation Time: 5 minutes

Cooking Time: 0 minutes

Servings: 4

Ingredients:

For salad:

3 cups cooked whole-wheat fusilli 2 cups cherry tomatoes, halved

½ cup vegan cheese, shredded 4 cups spinach, chopped

2 cups edamame, thawed

1   large red onion, finely chopped

For dressing:

2   tablespoons white wine vinegar

½ teaspoon dried dill

2 tbsp e.v.o. oil Salt to taste

Pepper to taste

Directions:

To make the dressing:

1.   Add the ingredients and mix well. Set aside for a while for the flavors to set in.

To make the salad:

2.   Add all the ingredients of the salad to a bowl. Toss well.

3.   Drizzle dressing on top. Toss well.

4.   Divide into 4 plates and serve.

Nutrition:

Calories: 684 Fat: 33.6g Carbs: 69.5g Protein: 31.7g

Italian Veggie Salad

Preparation Time: 10 minutes

Cooking Time: 0 minutes

Servings: 8

Ingredients:

For salad:

1 cup fresh baby carrots, quartered lengthwise 1 celery rib, sliced

3 large mushrooms, thinly sliced

1 cup cauliflower florets, bite-sized, blanched 1 cup broccoli florets, blanched

1 cup thinly sliced radish

4-5 oz. hearts of romaine salad mix to serve

For dressing:

½ package Italian salad dressing mix 3 tablespoons white vinegar

3 tablespoons water

3 tablespoons olive oil

3-4 pepperoncino, chopped

Directions:

To make the salad:

1.   Add all the ingredients of the salad except hearts of romaine to a bowl and toss.

To make the dressing:

2.   Add all the ingredients of the dressing in a small bowl. Whisk well.

3.   Pour dressing over salad and toss well. Refrigerate for a couple of hours.

4.   Place romaine in a large bowl. Place the chilled salad over it and serve.

Nutrition: Calories: 84 Fat: 6.7g Carbs: 5g Protein: 2g

Glazed Carrots

Prep Time: 12 minutes Cooking Time: 8 minutes
Servings: 4

Ingredients:

1-pound baby carrots peeled 1 tablespoon Maple syrup

1 tablespoon olive oil

1 teaspoon coriander, ground 1/2 teaspoon minced
garlic

1 teaspoon turmeric powder

1 tablespoon apple cider vinegar 1 tablespoon sesame
seeds

1/2 cup of water

Directions:

1.   Mix carrots and maple syrup and the other
ingredients, toss and leave aside for 10 minutes.

2.   Transfer the mix to the instant pot. Add water and
cook on Manual mode (High pressure) for 8 minutes.

3. Then make quick pressure release.

4. Transfer the mix to the serving bowls and serve.

Nutrition: Calories: 172, Fat: 4.9g, Fiber: 1.5g, Carbs: 6.1g, Protein: 4.3g

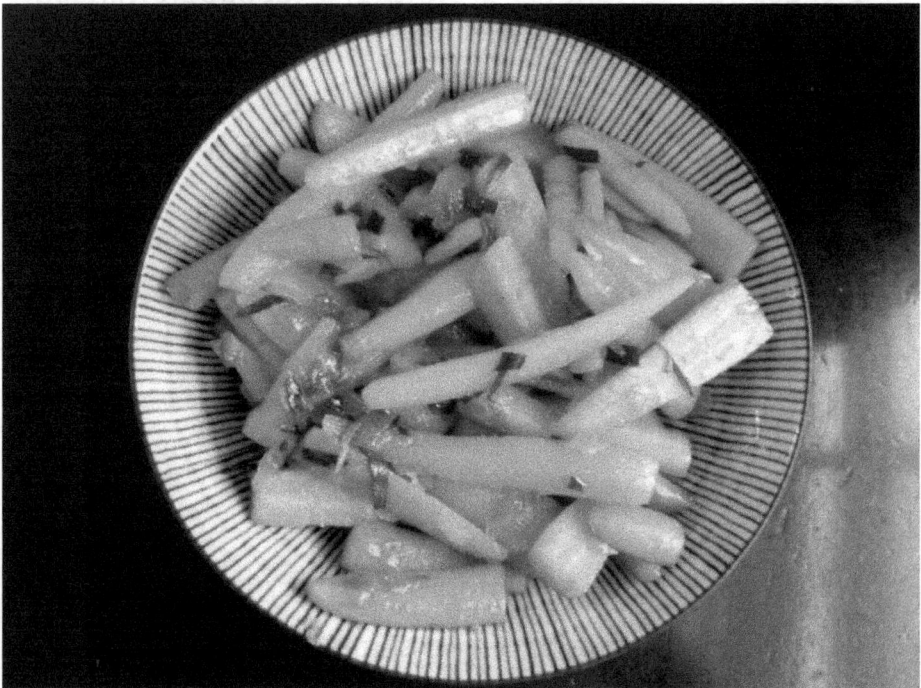

Broccoli Puree

Preparation Time: 15 minutes

Cooking Time: 15 minutes

Servings: 6

Ingredients:

1-pound broccoli florets 1/3 cup almond milk

1 cup of water

1 teaspoon dried oregano

1/2 teaspoon coriander, ground

Directions:

1.   Put the broccoli and the water in the instant pot and close the lid.

2.   Cook on Manual mode (High pressure) for 15 minutes. Use natural pressure release for 10 minutes.

3.   Strain, transfer to the food processor, add the rest of the ingredients, and pulse.

4.   Divide between plates and serve.

Nutrition: Calories: 182, Fat: 3.8g, Fiber: 4.8g, Carbs: 11.1g, Protein: 2g

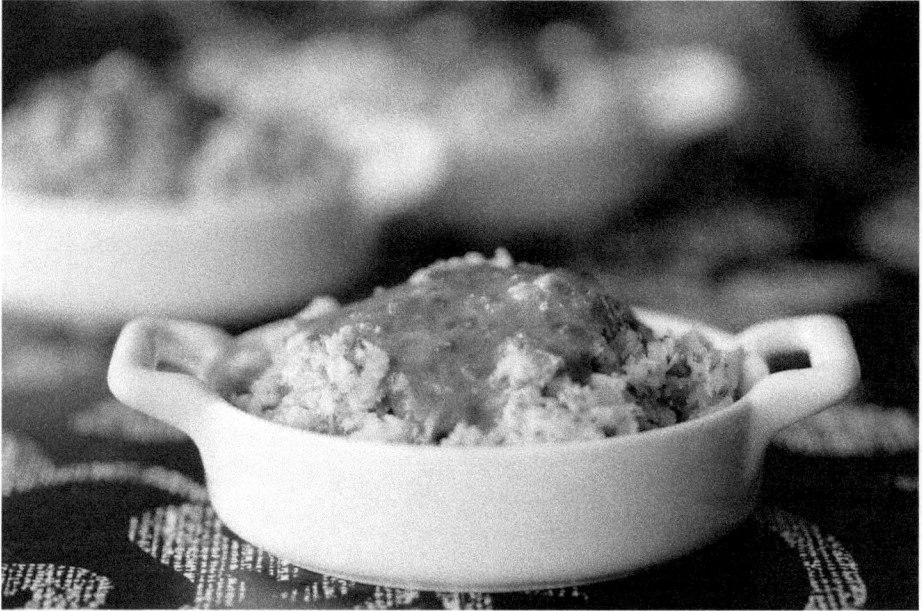

www.ingramcontent.com/pod-product-compliance
Lightning Source LLC
Chambersburg PA
CBHW050759030426
42336CB00012B/1872